LOG BOOK 1

LOG START DATE		LOG END DATE	
CONTINUED FROM LOG			

NAME	
ADDRESS	
EMAIL	
PHONE	
FAX	

NOTES

PERSONAL INFORMATION

NAME:	
D.O.B	
PHONE:	
ADDRESS:	
EMAIL:	
ALLERGIES	

INSURANCE INFORMATION

COMPANY:			
COVER DETAILS:			
START DATE		END DATE	
PHONE:			
EMAIL:			
ADDRESS			

EMERGENCY CONTACTS 1

Name:	**Name:**
Contact Number:	Relationship:

EMERGENCY CONTACT 2

Name:	**Name:**
Contact Number:	Relationship:

EMERGENCY CONTACTS 3

Name:	**Name:**
Contact Number:	Relationship:

NOTES

SPECIALIST CONTACTS

Name	
Specialist Type	
Contact Number	
Address	
Name	
Specialist Type	
Contact Number	
Address	
Name	
Specialist Type	
Contact Number	
Address	
Name	
Specialist Type	
Contact Number	
Address	

OTHERS / NOTES

MEDICATION TRACKER

Medicine

No	Medicine	Dose	Start Date	End Date	Frequency

Regular Medication

Medication	Date Started	Date Ended	Dose	Shape	Color
Special Instruction					

Medication	Date Started	Date Ended	Dose	Shape
Special Instruction				

Medication	Date Started	Date Ended	Dose	Shape	Color
Special Instruction					

Medication	Date Started	Date Ended	Dose	Shape
Special Instruction				

Medication	Date Started	Date Ended	Dose	Shape	Color
Special Instruction					

Medication	Date Started	Date Ended	Dose	Shape
Special Instruction				

Medication	Date Started	Date Ended	Dose	Shape	Color
Special Instruction					

Medication	Date Started	Date Ended	Dose	Shape
Special Instruction				

Medication	Date Started	Date Ended	Dose	Shape	Color
Special Instruction					

MEDICAL HISTORY

	YES	NO	NOTES
High Blood Pressure			
Stroke			
High Cholesterol			
Diabetes			
Glaucoma			
Epilepsy			
Asthma			
Obesity			
Allergies			
Cancer (type)			
Hearing Loss			
Alcohol Misuse			
Drug Misuse			
Kidney Problems			
Incontinent			
Ambulant			

IMPORTANT MEDICAL HISTORY

CAREGIVER DETAILS

NAME: _____
COMPANY: _____
RELATIONSHIP: _____
CONTACT No.: _____
EMAIL: _____
ADDRESS: _____
_____

VISITS: ○ Physical ○ Phone ○ Email

FREQUENCY
○ Daily ○ Weekly ○ Fortnightly
○ Monthly

TYPE OF ASSISTANCE ○ Personal Care
○ Cleaning ○ Meal Prep. ○ Medication
○ Medical Appointments ○ Transportation
○ Bill Paying ○ Shopping ○ Prompting
○ Other _____

NAME: _____
COMPANY: _____
RELATIONSHIP: _____
CONTACT No.: _____
EMAIL: _____
ADDRESS: _____
_____

VISITS: ○ Physical ○ Phone ○ Email

FREQUENCY
○ Daily ○ Weekly ○ Fortnightly
○ Monthly

TYPE OF ASSISTANCE ○ Personal Care
○ Cleaning ○ Meal Prep. ○ Medication
○ Medical Appointments ○ Transportation
○ Bill Paying ○ Shopping ○ Prompting
○ Other _____

Other Information
_____
_____
_____
_____
_____

CAREGIVER DETAILS

NAME:
COMPANY:
RELATIONSHIP:
CONTACT No.:
EMAIL:
ADDRESS:

VISITS: ○ Physical ○ Phone ○ Email

FREQUENCY
○ Daily ○ Weekly ○ Fortnightly
○ Monthly

TYPE OF ASSISTANCE ○ Personal Care
○ Cleaning ○ Meal Prep. ○ Medication
○ Medical Appointments ○ Transportation
○ Bill Paying ○ Shopping ○ Prompting
○ Other _____

NAME:
COMPANY:
RELATIONSHIP:
CONTACT No.:
EMAIL:
ADDRESS:

VISITS: ○ Physical ○ Phone ○ Email

FREQUENCY
○ Daily ○ Weekly ○ Fortnightly
○ Monthly

TYPE OF ASSISTANCE ○ Personal Care
○ Cleaning ○ Meal Prep. ○ Medication
○ Medical Appointments ○ Transportation
○ Bill Paying ○ Shopping ○ Prompting
○ Other _____

Other Information
_____
_____
_____
_____
_____

CAREGIVER DETAILS

NAME:
COMPANY:
RELATIONSHIP:
CONTACT No.:
EMAIL:
ADDRESS:

VISITS: ○ Physical ○ Phone ○ Email

FREQUENCY
○ Daily ○ Weekly ○ Fortnightly
○ Monthly

TYPE OF ASSISTANCE ○ Personal Care
○ Cleaning ○ Meal Prep. ○ Medication
○ Medical Appointments ○ Transportation
○ Bill Paying ○ Shopping ○ Prompting
○ Other _____

NAME:
COMPANY:
RELATIONSHIP:
CONTACT No.:
EMAIL:
ADDRESS:

VISITS: ○ Physical ○ Phone ○ Email

FREQUENCY
○ Daily ○ Weekly ○ Fortnightly
○ Monthly

TYPE OF ASSISTANCE ○ Personal Care
○ Cleaning ○ Meal Prep. ○ Medication
○ Medical Appointments ○ Transportation
○ Bill Paying ○ Shopping ○ Prompting
○ Other _____

Other Information

_____
_____
_____
_____
_____

CAREGIVER DETAILS

NAME:
COMPANY:
RELATIONSHIP:
CONTACT No.:
EMAIL:
ADDRESS:

VISITS: ○ Physical ○ Phone ○ Email

FREQUENCY
○ Daily ○ Weekly ○ Fortnightly
○ Monthly

TYPE OF ASSISTANCE ○ Personal Care
○ Cleaning ○ Meal Prep. ○ Medication
○ Medical Appointments ○ Transportation
○ Bill Paying ○ Shopping ○ Prompting
○ Other _____

NAME:
COMPANY:
RELATIONSHIP:
CONTACT No.:
EMAIL:
ADDRESS:

VISITS: ○ Physical ○ Phone ○ Email

FREQUENCY
○ Daily ○ Weekly ○ Fortnightly
○ Monthly

TYPE OF ASSISTANCE ○ Personal Care
○ Cleaning ○ Meal Prep. ○ Medication
○ Medical Appointments ○ Transportation
○ Bill Paying ○ Shopping ○ Prompting
○ Other _____

Other Information
_____
_____
_____
_____
_____

CAREGIVER SCHEDULE

CARER NAME: **DATE/ WEEK**

🕐	Sunday	Monday	Tuesday	Wednesday	Thursday	Friday	Saturday

CARER NAME: **DATE/ WEEK**

🕐	Sunday	Monday	Tuesday	Wednesday	Thursday	Friday	Saturday

CARER NAME: **DATE/ WEEK**

🕐	Sunday	Monday	Tuesday	Wednesday	Thursday	Friday	Saturday

CARER NAME: **DATE/ WEEK**

🕐	Sunday	Monday	Tuesday	Wednesday	Thursday	Friday	Saturday

CAREGIVER SCHEDULE

CARER NAME: **DATE/ WEEK**

🕒	Sunday	Monday	Tuesday	Wednesday	Thursday	Friday	Saturday

CARER NAME: **DATE/ WEEK**

🕒	Sunday	Monday	Tuesday	Wednesday	Thursday	Friday	Saturday

CARER NAME: **DATE/ WEEK**

🕒	Sunday	Monday	Tuesday	Wednesday	Thursday	Friday	Saturday

CARER NAME: **DATE/ WEEK**

🕒	Sunday	Monday	Tuesday	Wednesday	Thursday	Friday	Saturday

CAREGIVER SCHEDULE

CARER NAME: **DATE/ WEEK**

🕐	Sunday	Monday	Tuesday	Wednesday	Thursday	Friday	Saturday

CARER NAME: **DATE/ WEEK**

🕐	Sunday	Monday	Tuesday	Wednesday	Thursday	Friday	Saturday

CARER NAME: **DATE/ WEEK**

🕐	Sunday	Monday	Tuesday	Wednesday	Thursday	Friday	Saturday

CARER NAME: **DATE/ WEEK**

🕐	Sunday	Monday	Tuesday	Wednesday	Thursday	Friday	Saturday

CAREGIVER SCHEDULE

CARER NAME: **DATE/ WEEK**

🕐	Sunday	Monday	Tuesday	Wednesday	Thursday	Friday	Saturday

CARER NAME: **DATE/ WEEK**

🕐	Sunday	Monday	Tuesday	Wednesday	Thursday	Friday	Saturday

CARER NAME: **DATE/ WEEK**

🕐	Sunday	Monday	Tuesday	Wednesday	Thursday	Friday	Saturday

CARER NAME: **DATE/ WEEK**

🕐	Sunday	Monday	Tuesday	Wednesday	Thursday	Friday	Saturday

CAREGIVER SCHEDULE

CARER NAME: **DATE/ WEEK**

🕐	Sunday	Monday	Tuesday	Wednesday	Thursday	Friday	Saturday

CARER NAME: **DATE/ WEEK**

🕐	Sunday	Monday	Tuesday	Wednesday	Thursday	Friday	Saturday

CARER NAME: **DATE/ WEEK**

🕐	Sunday	Monday	Tuesday	Wednesday	Thursday	Friday	Saturday

CARER NAME: **DATE/ WEEK**

🕐	Sunday	Monday	Tuesday	Wednesday	Thursday	Friday	Saturday

CAREGIVER SCHEDULE

CARER NAME: **DATE/ WEEK**

🕐	Sunday	Monday	Tuesday	Wednesday	Thursday	Friday	Saturday

CARER NAME: **DATE/ WEEK**

🕐	Sunday	Monday	Tuesday	Wednesday	Thursday	Friday	Saturday

CARER NAME: **DATE/ WEEK**

🕐	Sunday	Monday	Tuesday	Wednesday	Thursday	Friday	Saturday

CARER NAME: **DATE/ WEEK**

🕐	Sunday	Monday	Tuesday	Wednesday	Thursday	Friday	Saturday

SELF-CARE ABILITIES

PERSONAL CARE	YES	NO	NOTES
Bathing			
Brush Teeth			
Change Clothes			
Shoes On/Off			
Mobility			
Toileting			
Eating			
Walking			

HOME CARE	YES	NO	NOTES
Meal Prep			
Laundry			
Shopping			
Cleaning			
Transport			

	YES	NO	NOTES

SELF-CARE ABILITIES

PHONE CALL LOG

Name of Person/Company Called	Date	Time	Phone Number	Message / Reason for call	Follow-Up Notes

PHONE CALL LOG

Name of Person/Company Called	Date	Time	Phone Number	Message / Reason for call	Follow-Up Notes

PHONE CALL LOG

Name of Person/Company Called	Date	Time	Phone Number	Message / Reason for call	Follow-Up Notes

PHONE CALL LOG

Name of Person/Company Called	Date	Time	Phone Number	Message / Reason for call	Follow-Up Notes

PHONE CALL LOG

Name of Person/Company Called	Date	Time	Phone Number	Message / Reason for call	Follow-Up Notes

PHONE CALL LOG

Name of Person/Company Called	Date	Time	Phone Number	Message / Reason for call	Follow-Up Notes

Name of Person/Company Called	Date	Time	Phone Number	Message / Reason for call	Follow-Up Notes

PHONE CALL LOG

CARE LOG

DATE		CARER	
START TIME		TIME ENDED	

MEDICATION	DOSE	TIME	NOTES

MEALS		TIME	QUANTITY
Breakfast			
Lunch			
Dinner			
Snack			
Snack			

TIME	ACTIVITIES	NAPS	TIME	TIME UP

PERSONAL HYGIENE	TIME	NOTES

SUPPLIES NEEDED	PURCHASED	DETAILS

SUMMARY OF DUTIES DONE & ANY CONCERNS

CARE LOG

DATE		CARER	
START TIME		TIME ENDED	

MEDICATION	DOSE	TIME	NOTES

MEALS		TIME	QUANTITY
Breakfast			
Lunch			
Dinner			
Snack			
Snack			

TIME	ACTIVITIES	NAPS	TIME	TIME UP

PERSONAL HYGIENE	TIME	NOTES

SUPPLIES NEEDED	PURCHASED	DETAILS

SUMMARY OF DUTIES DONE & ANY CONCERNS

CARE LOG

DATE		CARER	
START TIME		TIME ENDED	

MEDICATION	DOSE	TIME	NOTES

MEALS		TIME	QUANTITY
Breakfast			
Lunch			
Dinner			
Snack			
Snack			

TIME	ACTIVITIES	NAPS	TIME	TIME UP

PERSONAL HYGIENE	TIME	NOTES

SUPPLIES NEEDED	PURCHASED	DETAILS

SUMMARY OF DUTIES DONE & ANY CONCERNS

CARE LOG

DATE		CARER	
START TIME		TIME ENDED	

MEDICATION	DOSE	TIME	NOTES

MEALS		TIME	QUANTITY
Breakfast			
Lunch			
Dinner			
Snack			
Snack			

TIME	ACTIVITIES	NAPS	TIME	TIME UP

PERSONAL HYGIENE	TIME	NOTES

SUPPLIES NEEDED	PURCHASED	DETAILS

SUMMARY OF DUTIES DONE & ANY CONCERNS

CARE LOG

DATE		CARER	
START TIME		TIME ENDED	

MEDICATION	DOSE	TIME	NOTES

MEALS		TIME	QUANTITY
Breakfast			
Lunch			
Dinner			
Snack			
Snack			

TIME	ACTIVITIES	NAPS	TIME	TIME UP

PERSONAL HYGIENE	TIME	NOTES

SUPPLIES NEEDED	PURCHASED	DETAILS

SUMMARY OF DUTIES DONE & ANY CONCERNS

CARE LOG

DATE		CARER	
START TIME		TIME ENDED	

MEDICATION	DOSE	TIME	NOTES

MEALS		TIME	QUANTITY
Breakfast			
Lunch			
Dinner			
Snack			
Snack			

TIME	ACTIVITIES	NAPS	TIME	TIME UP

PERSONAL HYGIENE	TIME	NOTES

SUPPLIES NEEDED	PURCHASED	DETAILS

SUMMARY OF DUTIES DONE & ANY CONCERNS

CARE LOG

DATE		CARER	
START TIME		TIME ENDED	

MEDICATION	DOSE	TIME	NOTES

MEALS		TIME	QUANTITY
Breakfast			
Lunch			
Dinner			
Snack			
Snack			

TIME	ACTIVITIES		TIME	TIME UP
		NAPS		

PERSONAL HYGIENE	TIME	NOTES

SUPPLIES NEEDED	PURCHASED	DETAILS

SUMMARY OF DUTIES DONE & ANY CONCERNS

CARE LOG

DATE		CARER	
START TIME		TIME ENDED	

MEDICATION	DOSE	TIME	NOTES

MEALS		TIME	QUANTITY
Breakfast			
Lunch			
Dinner			
Snack			
Snack			

TIME	ACTIVITIES	NAPS	TIME	TIME UP

PERSONAL HYGIENE	TIME	NOTES

SUPPLIES NEEDED	PURCHASED	DETAILS

SUMMARY OF DUTIES DONE & ANY CONCERNS

CARE LOG

DATE		CARER	
START TIME		TIME ENDED	

MEDICATION	DOSE	TIME	NOTES

MEALS		TIME	QUANTITY
Breakfast			
Lunch			
Dinner			
Snack			
Snack			

TIME	ACTIVITIES	NAPS	TIME	TIME UP

PERSONAL HYGIENE	TIME	NOTES

SUPPLIES NEEDED	PURCHASED	DETAILS

SUMMARY OF DUTIES DONE & ANY CONCERNS

CARE LOG

DATE		CARER	
START TIME		TIME ENDED	

MEDICATION	DOSE	TIME	NOTES

MEALS		TIME	QUANTITY
Breakfast			
Lunch			
Dinner			
Snack			
Snack			

TIME	ACTIVITIES	NAPS	TIME	TIME UP

PERSONAL HYGIENE	TIME	NOTES

SUPPLIES NEEDED	PURCHASED	DETAILS

SUMMARY OF DUTIES DONE & ANY CONCERNS

CARE LOG

DATE		CARER	
START TIME		TIME ENDED	

MEDICATION	DOSE	TIME	NOTES

MEALS		TIME	QUANTITY
Breakfast			
Lunch			
Dinner			
Snack			
Snack			

TIME	ACTIVITIES	NAPS	TIME	TIME UP

PERSONAL HYGIENE	TIME	NOTES

SUPPLIES NEEDED	PURCHASED	DETAILS

SUMMARY OF DUTIES DONE & ANY CONCERNS

CARE LOG

DATE		CARER	
START TIME		TIME ENDED	

MEDICATION	DOSE	TIME	NOTES

MEALS		TIME	QUANTITY
Breakfast			
Lunch			
Dinner			
Snack			
Snack			

TIME	ACTIVITIES	NAPS	TIME	TIME UP

PERSONAL HYGIENE	TIME	NOTES

SUPPLIES NEEDED	PURCHASED	DETAILS

SUMMARY OF DUTIES DONE & ANY CONCERNS

CARE LOG

DATE		CARER	
START TIME		TIME ENDED	

MEDICATION	DOSE	TIME	NOTES

MEALS		TIME	QUANTITY
Breakfast			
Lunch			
Dinner			
Snack			
Snack			

TIME	ACTIVITIES	NAPS	TIME	TIME UP

PERSONAL HYGIENE	TIME	NOTES

SUPPLIES NEEDED	PURCHASED	DETAILS

SUMMARY OF DUTIES DONE & ANY CONCERNS

CARE LOG

DATE		CARER	
START TIME		TIME ENDED	

MEDICATION	DOSE	TIME	NOTES

MEALS		TIME	QUANTITY
Breakfast			
Lunch			
Dinner			
Snack			
Snack			

TIME	ACTIVITIES	NAPS	TIME	TIME UP

PERSONAL HYGIENE	TIME	NOTES

SUPPLIES NEEDED	PURCHASED	DETAILS

SUMMARY OF DUTIES DONE & ANY CONCERNS

CARE LOG

DATE		CARER	
START TIME		TIME ENDED	

MEDICATION	DOSE	TIME	NOTES

MEALS		TIME	QUANTITY
Breakfast			
Lunch			
Dinner			
Snack			
Snack			

TIME	ACTIVITIES	NAPS	TIME	TIME UP

PERSONAL HYGIENE	TIME	NOTES

SUPPLIES NEEDED	PURCHASED	DETAILS

SUMMARY OF DUTIES DONE & ANY CONCERNS

CARE LOG

DATE		CARER	
START TIME		TIME ENDED	

MEDICATION	DOSE	TIME	NOTES

MEALS		TIME	QUANTITY
Breakfast			
Lunch			
Dinner			
Snack			
Snack			

TIME	ACTIVITIES	NAPS	TIME	TIME UP

PERSONAL HYGIENE	TIME	NOTES

SUPPLIES NEEDED	PURCHASED	DETAILS

SUMMARY OF DUTIES DONE & ANY CONCERNS

CARE LOG

DATE		CARER	
START TIME		TIME ENDED	

MEDICATION	DOSE	TIME	NOTES

MEALS		TIME	QUANTITY
Breakfast			
Lunch			
Dinner			
Snack			
Snack			

TIME	ACTIVITIES	NAPS	TIME	TIME UP

PERSONAL HYGIENE	TIME	NOTES

SUPPLIES NEEDED	PURCHASED	DETAILS

SUMMARY OF DUTIES DONE & ANY CONCERNS

CARE LOG

DATE		CARER	
START TIME		TIME ENDED	

MEDICATION	DOSE	TIME	NOTES

MEALS		TIME	QUANTITY
Breakfast			
Lunch			
Dinner			
Snack			
Snack			

TIME	ACTIVITIES	NAPS	TIME	TIME UP

PERSONAL HYGIENE	TIME	NOTES

SUPPLIES NEEDED	PURCHASED	DETAILS

SUMMARY OF DUTIES DONE & ANY CONCERNS

CARE LOG

DATE		CARER	
START TIME		TIME ENDED	

MEDICATION	DOSE	TIME	NOTES

MEALS		TIME	QUANTITY
Breakfast			
Lunch			
Dinner			
Snack			
Snack			

TIME	ACTIVITIES	NAPS	TIME	TIME UP

PERSONAL HYGIENE	TIME	NOTES

SUPPLIES NEEDED	PURCHASED	DETAILS

SUMMARY OF DUTIES DONE & ANY CONCERNS

_____
_____
_____
_____
_____

CARE LOG

DATE		CARER	
START TIME		TIME ENDED	

MEDICATION	DOSE	TIME	NOTES

MEALS		TIME	QUANTITY
Breakfast			
Lunch			
Dinner			
Snack			
Snack			

TIME	ACTIVITIES	NAPS	TIME	TIME UP

PERSONAL HYGIENE	TIME	NOTES

SUPPLIES NEEDED	PURCHASED	DETAILS

SUMMARY OF DUTIES DONE & ANY CONCERNS

CARE LOG

DATE		CARER	
START TIME		TIME ENDED	

MEDICATION	DOSE	TIME	NOTES

MEALS		TIME	QUANTITY
Breakfast			
Lunch			
Dinner			
Snack			
Snack			

TIME	ACTIVITIES	NAPS	TIME	TIME UP

PERSONAL HYGIENE	TIME	NOTES

SUPPLIES NEEDED	PURCHASED	DETAILS

SUMMARY OF DUTIES DONE & ANY CONCERNS

CARE LOG

DATE		CARER	
START TIME		TIME ENDED	

MEDICATION	DOSE	TIME	NOTES

MEALS		TIME	QUANTITY
Breakfast			
Lunch			
Dinner			
Snack			
Snack			

TIME	ACTIVITIES	NAPS	TIME	TIME UP

PERSONAL HYGIENE	TIME	NOTES

SUPPLIES NEEDED	PURCHASED	DETAILS

SUMMARY OF DUTIES DONE & ANY CONCERNS

CARE LOG

DATE		CARER	
START TIME		TIME ENDED	

MEDICATION	DOSE	TIME	NOTES

MEALS		TIME	QUANTITY
Breakfast			
Lunch			
Dinner			
Snack			
Snack			

TIME	ACTIVITIES	NAPS	TIME	TIME UP

PERSONAL HYGIENE	TIME	NOTES

SUPPLIES NEEDED	PURCHASED	DETAILS

SUMMARY OF DUTIES DONE & ANY CONCERNS

_____
_____
_____
_____
_____

CARE LOG

DATE		CARER	
START TIME		TIME ENDED	

MEDICATION	DOSE	TIME	NOTES

MEALS		TIME	QUANTITY
Breakfast			
Lunch			
Dinner			
Snack			
Snack			

TIME	ACTIVITIES	NAPS	TIME	TIME UP

PERSONAL HYGIENE	TIME	NOTES

SUPPLIES NEEDED	PURCHASED	DETAILS

SUMMARY OF DUTIES DONE & ANY CONCERNS

CARE LOG

DATE		CARER	
START TIME		TIME ENDED	

MEDICATION	DOSE	TIME	NOTES

MEALS		TIME	QUANTITY
Breakfast			
Lunch			
Dinner			
Snack			
Snack			

TIME	ACTIVITIES	NAPS	TIME	TIME UP

PERSONAL HYGIENE	TIME	NOTES

SUPPLIES NEEDED	PURCHASED	DETAILS

SUMMARY OF DUTIES DONE & ANY CONCERNS

CARE LOG

DATE		CARER	
START TIME		TIME ENDED	

MEDICATION	DOSE	TIME	NOTES

MEALS		TIME	QUANTITY
Breakfast			
Lunch			
Dinner			
Snack			
Snack			

TIME	ACTIVITIES	NAPS	TIME	TIME UP

PERSONAL HYGIENE	TIME	NOTES

SUPPLIES NEEDED	PURCHASED	DETAILS

SUMMARY OF DUTIES DONE & ANY CONCERNS

CARE LOG

DATE		CARER	
START TIME		TIME ENDED	

MEDICATION	DOSE	TIME	NOTES

MEALS		TIME	QUANTITY
Breakfast			
Lunch			
Dinner			
Snack			
Snack			

TIME	ACTIVITIES	NAPS	TIME	TIME UP

PERSONAL HYGIENE	TIME	NOTES

SUPPLIES NEEDED	PURCHASED	DETAILS

SUMMARY OF DUTIES DONE & ANY CONCERNS

_____
_____
_____
_____
_____
_____

CARE LOG

DATE		CARER	
START TIME		TIME ENDED	

MEDICATION	DOSE	TIME	NOTES

MEALS		TIME	QUANTITY
Breakfast			
Lunch			
Dinner			
Snack			
Snack			

TIME	ACTIVITIES	NAPS	TIME	TIME UP

PERSONAL HYGIENE	TIME	NOTES

SUPPLIES NEEDED	PURCHASED	DETAILS

SUMMARY OF DUTIES DONE & ANY CONCERNS

CARE LOG

DATE		CARER	
START TIME		TIME ENDED	

MEDICATION	DOSE	TIME	NOTES

MEALS		TIME	QUANTITY
Breakfast			
Lunch			
Dinner			
Snack			
Snack			

TIME	ACTIVITIES	NAPS	TIME	TIME UP

PERSONAL HYGIENE	TIME	NOTES

SUPPLIES NEEDED	PURCHASED	DETAILS

SUMMARY OF DUTIES DONE & ANY CONCERNS

CARE LOG

DATE		CARER	
START TIME		TIME ENDED	

MEDICATION	DOSE	TIME	NOTES

MEALS		TIME	QUANTITY
Breakfast			
Lunch			
Dinner			
Snack			
Snack			

TIME	ACTIVITIES	NAPS	TIME	TIME UP

PERSONAL HYGIENE	TIME	NOTES

SUPPLIES NEEDED	PURCHASED	DETAILS

SUMMARY OF DUTIES DONE & ANY CONCERNS

_____
_____
_____
_____
_____

CARE LOG

DATE		CARER	
START TIME		TIME ENDED	

MEDICATION	DOSE	TIME	NOTES

MEALS		TIME	QUANTITY
Breakfast			
Lunch			
Dinner			
Snack			
Snack			

TIME	ACTIVITIES	NAPS	TIME	TIME UP

PERSONAL HYGIENE	TIME	NOTES

SUPPLIES NEEDED	PURCHASED	DETAILS

SUMMARY OF DUTIES DONE & ANY CONCERNS

CARE LOG

DATE		CARER	
START TIME		TIME ENDED	

MEDICATION	DOSE	TIME	NOTES

MEALS		TIME	QUANTITY
Breakfast			
Lunch			
Dinner			
Snack			
Snack			

TIME	ACTIVITIES	NAPS	TIME	TIME UP

PERSONAL HYGIENE	TIME	NOTES

SUPPLIES NEEDED	PURCHASED	DETAILS

SUMMARY OF DUTIES DONE & ANY CONCERNS

_____

_____

_____

_____

CARE LOG

DATE		CARER	
START TIME		TIME ENDED	

MEDICATION	DOSE	TIME	NOTES

MEALS		TIME	QUANTITY
Breakfast			
Lunch			
Dinner			
Snack			
Snack			

TIME	ACTIVITIES	NAPS	TIME	TIME UP

PERSONAL HYGIENE	TIME	NOTES

SUPPLIES NEEDED	PURCHASED	DETAILS

SUMMARY OF DUTIES DONE & ANY CONCERNS

CARE LOG

DATE		CARER	
START TIME		TIME ENDED	

MEDICATION	DOSE	TIME	NOTES

MEALS		TIME	QUANTITY
Breakfast			
Lunch			
Dinner			
Snack			
Snack			

TIME	ACTIVITIES	NAPS	TIME	TIME UP

PERSONAL HYGIENE	TIME	NOTES

SUPPLIES NEEDED	PURCHASED	DETAILS

SUMMARY OF DUTIES DONE & ANY CONCERNS

CARE LOG

DATE		CARER	
START TIME		TIME ENDED	

MEDICATION	DOSE	TIME	NOTES

MEALS		TIME	QUANTITY
Breakfast			
Lunch			
Dinner			
Snack			
Snack			

TIME	ACTIVITIES	NAPS	TIME	TIME UP

PERSONAL HYGIENE	TIME	NOTES

SUPPLIES NEEDED	PURCHASED	DETAILS

SUMMARY OF DUTIES DONE & ANY CONCERNS

CARE LOG

DATE		CARER	
START TIME		TIME ENDED	

MEDICATION	DOSE	TIME	NOTES

MEALS		TIME	QUANTITY
Breakfast			
Lunch			
Dinner			
Snack			
Snack			

TIME	ACTIVITIES	NAPS	TIME	TIME UP

PERSONAL HYGIENE	TIME	NOTES

SUPPLIES NEEDED	PURCHASED	DETAILS

SUMMARY OF DUTIES DONE & ANY CONCERNS

CARE LOG

DATE		CARER	
START TIME		TIME ENDED	

MEDICATION	DOSE	TIME	NOTES

MEALS		TIME	QUANTITY
Breakfast			
Lunch			
Dinner			
Snack			
Snack			

TIME	ACTIVITIES	NAPS	TIME	TIME UP

PERSONAL HYGIENE	TIME	NOTES

SUPPLIES NEEDED	PURCHASED	DETAILS

SUMMARY OF DUTIES DONE & ANY CONCERNS

CARE LOG

DATE		CARER	
START TIME		TIME ENDED	

MEDICATION	DOSE	TIME	NOTES

MEALS		TIME	QUANTITY
Breakfast			
Lunch			
Dinner			
Snack			
Snack			

TIME	ACTIVITIES	NAPS	TIME	TIME UP

PERSONAL HYGIENE	TIME	NOTES

SUPPLIES NEEDED	PURCHASED	DETAILS

SUMMARY OF DUTIES DONE & ANY CONCERNS

CARE LOG

DATE		CARER	
START TIME		TIME ENDED	

MEDICATION	DOSE	TIME	NOTES

MEALS		TIME	QUANTITY
Breakfast			
Lunch			
Dinner			
Snack			
Snack			

TIME	ACTIVITIES	NAPS	TIME	TIME UP

PERSONAL HYGIENE	TIME	NOTES

SUPPLIES NEEDED	PURCHASED	DETAILS

SUMMARY OF DUTIES DONE & ANY CONCERNS

CARE LOG

DATE		CARER	
START TIME		TIME ENDED	

MEDICATION	DOSE	TIME	NOTES

MEALS		TIME	QUANTITY
Breakfast			
Lunch			
Dinner			
Snack			
Snack			

TIME	ACTIVITIES	NAPS	TIME	TIME UP

PERSONAL HYGIENE	TIME	NOTES

SUPPLIES NEEDED	PURCHASED	DETAILS

SUMMARY OF DUTIES DONE & ANY CONCERNS

_____
_____
_____
_____
_____

CARE LOG

DATE		CARER	
START TIME		TIME ENDED	

MEDICATION	DOSE	TIME	NOTES

MEALS		TIME	QUANTITY
Breakfast			
Lunch			
Dinner			
Snack			
Snack			

TIME	ACTIVITIES	NAPS	TIME	TIME UP

PERSONAL HYGIENE	TIME	NOTES

SUPPLIES NEEDED	PURCHASED	DETAILS

SUMMARY OF DUTIES DONE & ANY CONCERNS

CARE LOG

DATE		CARER	
START TIME		TIME ENDED	

MEDICATION	DOSE	TIME	NOTES

MEALS		TIME	QUANTITY
Breakfast			
Lunch			
Dinner			
Snack			
Snack			

TIME	ACTIVITIES	NAPS	TIME	TIME UP

PERSONAL HYGIENE	TIME	NOTES

SUPPLIES NEEDED	PURCHASED	DETAILS

SUMMARY OF DUTIES DONE & ANY CONCERNS

CARE LOG

DATE		CARER	
START TIME		TIME ENDED	

MEDICATION	DOSE	TIME	NOTES

MEALS		TIME	QUANTITY
Breakfast			
Lunch			
Dinner			
Snack			
Snack			

TIME	ACTIVITIES	NAPS	TIME	TIME UP

PERSONAL HYGIENE	TIME	NOTES

SUPPLIES NEEDED	PURCHASED	DETAILS

SUMMARY OF DUTIES DONE & ANY CONCERNS

CARE LOG

DATE		CARER	
START TIME		TIME ENDED	

MEDICATION	DOSE	TIME	NOTES

MEALS		TIME	QUANTITY
Breakfast			
Lunch			
Dinner			
Snack			
Snack			

TIME	ACTIVITIES	NAPS	TIME	TIME UP

PERSONAL HYGIENE	TIME	NOTES

SUPPLIES NEEDED	PURCHASED	DETAILS

SUMMARY OF DUTIES DONE & ANY CONCERNS

_____
_____
_____
_____
_____

CARE LOG

DATE		CARER	
START TIME		TIME ENDED	

MEDICATION	DOSE	TIME	NOTES

MEALS		TIME	QUANTITY
Breakfast			
Lunch			
Dinner			
Snack			
Snack			

TIME	ACTIVITIES	NAPS	TIME	TIME UP

PERSONAL HYGIENE	TIME	NOTES

SUPPLIES NEEDED	PURCHASED	DETAILS

SUMMARY OF DUTIES DONE & ANY CONCERNS

CARE LOG

DATE		CARER	
START TIME		TIME ENDED	

MEDICATION	DOSE	TIME	NOTES

MEALS		TIME	QUANTITY
Breakfast			
Lunch			
Dinner			
Snack			
Snack			

TIME	ACTIVITIES	NAPS	TIME	TIME UP

PERSONAL HYGIENE	TIME	NOTES

SUPPLIES NEEDED	PURCHASED	DETAILS

SUMMARY OF DUTIES DONE & ANY CONCERNS

CARE LOG

DATE		CARER	
START TIME		TIME ENDED	

MEDICATION	DOSE	TIME	NOTES

MEALS		TIME	QUANTITY
Breakfast			
Lunch			
Dinner			
Snack			
Snack			

TIME	ACTIVITIES	NAPS	TIME	TIME UP

PERSONAL HYGIENE	TIME	NOTES

SUPPLIES NEEDED	PURCHASED	DETAILS

SUMMARY OF DUTIES DONE & ANY CONCERNS

_____
_____
_____
_____

CARE LOG

DATE		CARER	
START TIME		TIME ENDED	

MEDICATION	DOSE	TIME	NOTES

MEALS		TIME	QUANTITY
Breakfast			
Lunch			
Dinner			
Snack			
Snack			

TIME	ACTIVITIES	NAPS	TIME	TIME UP

PERSONAL HYGIENE	TIME	NOTES

SUPPLIES NEEDED	PURCHASED	DETAILS

SUMMARY OF DUTIES DONE & ANY CONCERNS

_____
_____
_____
_____
_____

CARE LOG

DATE		CARER	
START TIME		TIME ENDED	

MEDICATION	DOSE	TIME	NOTES

MEALS		TIME	QUANTITY
Breakfast			
Lunch			
Dinner			
Snack			
Snack			

TIME	ACTIVITIES	NAPS	TIME	TIME UP

PERSONAL HYGIENE	TIME	NOTES

SUPPLIES NEEDED	PURCHASED	DETAILS

SUMMARY OF DUTIES DONE & ANY CONCERNS

CARE LOG

DATE		CARER	
START TIME		TIME ENDED	

MEDICATION	DOSE	TIME	NOTES

MEALS		TIME	QUANTITY
Breakfast			
Lunch			
Dinner			
Snack			
Snack			

TIME	ACTIVITIES	NAPS	TIME	TIME UP

PERSONAL HYGIENE	TIME	NOTES

SUPPLIES NEEDED	PURCHASED	DETAILS

SUMMARY OF DUTIES DONE & ANY CONCERNS

_____

_____

_____

_____

_____

CARE LOG

DATE		CARER	
START TIME		TIME ENDED	

MEDICATION	DOSE	TIME	NOTES

MEALS		TIME	QUANTITY
Breakfast			
Lunch			
Dinner			
Snack			
Snack			

TIME	ACTIVITIES	NAPS	TIME	TIME UP

PERSONAL HYGIENE	TIME	NOTES

SUPPLIES NEEDED	PURCHASED	DETAILS

SUMMARY OF DUTIES DONE & ANY CONCERNS

CARE LOG

DATE		CARER	
START TIME		TIME ENDED	

MEDICATION	DOSE	TIME	NOTES

MEALS		TIME	QUANTITY
Breakfast			
Lunch			
Dinner			
Snack			
Snack			

TIME	ACTIVITIES	NAPS	TIME	TIME UP

PERSONAL HYGIENE	TIME	NOTES

SUPPLIES NEEDED	PURCHASED	DETAILS

SUMMARY OF DUTIES DONE & ANY CONCERNS

_____
_____
_____
_____
_____

CARE LOG

DATE		CARER	
START TIME		TIME ENDED	

MEDICATION	DOSE	TIME	NOTES

MEALS		TIME	QUANTITY
Breakfast			
Lunch			
Dinner			
Snack			
Snack			

TIME	ACTIVITIES	NAPS	TIME	TIME UP

PERSONAL HYGIENE	TIME	NOTES

SUPPLIES NEEDED	PURCHASED	DETAILS

SUMMARY OF DUTIES DONE & ANY CONCERNS

CARE LOG

DATE		CARER	
START TIME		TIME ENDED	

MEDICATION	DOSE	TIME	NOTES

MEALS		TIME	QUANTITY
Breakfast			
Lunch			
Dinner			
Snack			
Snack			

TIME	ACTIVITIES	NAPS	TIME	TIME UP

PERSONAL HYGIENE	TIME	NOTES

SUPPLIES NEEDED	PURCHASED	DETAILS

SUMMARY OF DUTIES DONE & ANY CONCERNS

_____
_____
_____
_____
_____

CARE LOG

DATE		CARER	
START TIME		TIME ENDED	

MEDICATION	DOSE	TIME	NOTES

MEALS		TIME	QUANTITY
Breakfast			
Lunch			
Dinner			
Snack			
Snack			

TIME	ACTIVITIES	NAPS	TIME	TIME UP

PERSONAL HYGIENE	TIME	NOTES

SUPPLIES NEEDED	PURCHASED	DETAILS

SUMMARY OF DUTIES DONE & ANY CONCERNS

CARE LOG

DATE		CARER	
START TIME		TIME ENDED	

MEDICATION	DOSE	TIME	NOTES

MEALS		TIME	QUANTITY
Breakfast			
Lunch			
Dinner			
Snack			
Snack			

TIME	ACTIVITIES	NAPS	TIME	TIME UP

PERSONAL HYGIENE	TIME	NOTES

SUPPLIES NEEDED	PURCHASED	DETAILS

SUMMARY OF DUTIES DONE & ANY CONCERNS

CARE LOG

DATE		CARER	
START TIME		TIME ENDED	

MEDICATION	DOSE	TIME	NOTES

MEALS		TIME	QUANTITY
Breakfast			
Lunch			
Dinner			
Snack			
Snack			

TIME	ACTIVITIES	NAPS	TIME	TIME UP

PERSONAL HYGIENE	TIME	NOTES

SUPPLIES NEEDED	PURCHASED	DETAILS

SUMMARY OF DUTIES DONE & ANY CONCERNS

CARE LOG

DATE		CARER	
START TIME		TIME ENDED	

MEDICATION	DOSE	TIME	NOTES

MEALS		TIME	QUANTITY
Breakfast			
Lunch			
Dinner			
Snack			
Snack			

TIME	ACTIVITIES	NAPS	TIME	TIME UP

PERSONAL HYGIENE	TIME	NOTES

SUPPLIES NEEDED	PURCHASED	DETAILS

SUMMARY OF DUTIES DONE & ANY CONCERNS

_____

_____

_____

_____

_____

CARE LOG

DATE		CARER	
START TIME		TIME ENDED	

MEDICATION	DOSE	TIME	NOTES

MEALS		TIME	QUANTITY
Breakfast			
Lunch			
Dinner			
Snack			
Snack			

TIME	ACTIVITIES	NAPS	TIME	TIME UP

PERSONAL HYGIENE	TIME	NOTES

SUPPLIES NEEDED	PURCHASED	DETAILS

SUMMARY OF DUTIES DONE & ANY CONCERNS

CARE LOG

DATE		CARER	
START TIME		TIME ENDED	

MEDICATION	DOSE	TIME	NOTES

MEALS		TIME	QUANTITY
Breakfast			
Lunch			
Dinner			
Snack			
Snack			

TIME	ACTIVITIES	NAPS	TIME	TIME UP

PERSONAL HYGIENE	TIME	NOTES

SUPPLIES NEEDED	PURCHASED	DETAILS

SUMMARY OF DUTIES DONE & ANY CONCERNS

_____
_____
_____
_____
_____

CARE LOG

DATE		CARER	
START TIME		TIME ENDED	

MEDICATION	DOSE	TIME	NOTES

MEALS		TIME	QUANTITY
Breakfast			
Lunch			
Dinner			
Snack			
Snack			

TIME	ACTIVITIES	NAPS	TIME	TIME UP

PERSONAL HYGIENE	TIME	NOTES

SUPPLIES NEEDED	PURCHASED	DETAILS

SUMMARY OF DUTIES DONE & ANY CONCERNS

CARE LOG

DATE		CARER	
START TIME		TIME ENDED	

MEDICATION	DOSE	TIME	NOTES

MEALS		TIME	QUANTITY
Breakfast			
Lunch			
Dinner			
Snack			
Snack			

TIME	ACTIVITIES	NAPS	TIME	TIME UP

PERSONAL HYGIENE	TIME	NOTES

SUPPLIES NEEDED	PURCHASED	DETAILS

SUMMARY OF DUTIES DONE & ANY CONCERNS

_____
_____
_____
_____
_____

CARE LOG

DATE		CARER	
START TIME		TIME ENDED	

MEDICATION	DOSE	TIME	NOTES

MEALS		TIME	QUANTITY
Breakfast			
Lunch			
Dinner			
Snack			
Snack			

TIME	ACTIVITIES	NAPS	TIME	TIME UP

PERSONAL HYGIENE	TIME	NOTES

SUPPLIES NEEDED	PURCHASED	DETAILS

SUMMARY OF DUTIES DONE & ANY CONCERNS

CARE LOG

DATE		CARER	
START TIME		**TIME ENDED**	

MEDICATION	DOSE	TIME	NOTES

MEALS		TIME	QUANTITY
Breakfast			
Lunch			
Dinner			
Snack			
Snack			

TIME	ACTIVITIES	NAPS	TIME	TIME UP

PERSONAL HYGIENE	TIME	NOTES

SUPPLIES NEEDED	PURCHASED	DETAILS

SUMMARY OF DUTIES DONE & ANY CONCERNS

_____
_____
_____
_____
_____

CARE LOG

DATE		CARER	
START TIME		TIME ENDED	

MEDICATION	DOSE	TIME	NOTES

MEALS		TIME	QUANTITY
Breakfast			
Lunch			
Dinner			
Snack			
Snack			

TIME	ACTIVITIES	NAPS	TIME	TIME UP

PERSONAL HYGIENE	TIME	NOTES

SUPPLIES NEEDED	PURCHASED	DETAILS

SUMMARY OF DUTIES DONE & ANY CONCERNS

CARE LOG

DATE		CARER	
START TIME		TIME ENDED	

MEDICATION	DOSE	TIME	NOTES

MEALS		TIME	QUANTITY
Breakfast			
Lunch			
Dinner			
Snack			
Snack			

TIME	ACTIVITIES	NAPS	TIME	TIME UP

PERSONAL HYGIENE	TIME	NOTES

SUPPLIES NEEDED	PURCHASED	DETAILS

SUMMARY OF DUTIES DONE & ANY CONCERNS

_____

_____

_____

_____

_____

CARE LOG

DATE		CARER	
START TIME		TIME ENDED	

MEDICATION	DOSE	TIME	NOTES

MEALS		TIME	QUANTITY
Breakfast			
Lunch			
Dinner			
Snack			
Snack			

TIME	ACTIVITIES	NAPS	TIME	TIME UP

PERSONAL HYGIENE	TIME	NOTES

SUPPLIES NEEDED	PURCHASED	DETAILS

SUMMARY OF DUTIES DONE & ANY CONCERNS

CARE LOG

DATE		CARER	
START TIME		TIME ENDED	

MEDICATION	DOSE	TIME	NOTES

MEALS		TIME	QUANTITY
Breakfast			
Lunch			
Dinner			
Snack			
Snack			

TIME	ACTIVITIES	NAPS	TIME	TIME UP

PERSONAL HYGIENE	TIME	NOTES

SUPPLIES NEEDED	PURCHASED	DETAILS

SUMMARY OF DUTIES DONE & ANY CONCERNS

_____
_____
_____
_____
_____

CARE LOG

DATE		CARER	
START TIME		TIME ENDED	

MEDICATION	DOSE	TIME	NOTES

MEALS		TIME	QUANTITY
Breakfast			
Lunch			
Dinner			
Snack			
Snack			

TIME	ACTIVITIES	NAPS	TIME	TIME UP

PERSONAL HYGIENE	TIME	NOTES

SUPPLIES NEEDED	PURCHASED	DETAILS

SUMMARY OF DUTIES DONE & ANY CONCERNS

CARE LOG

DATE		CARER	
START TIME		TIME ENDED	

MEDICATION	DOSE	TIME	NOTES

MEALS		TIME	QUANTITY
Breakfast			
Lunch			
Dinner			
Snack			
Snack			

TIME	ACTIVITIES	NAPS	TIME	TIME UP

PERSONAL HYGIENE	TIME	NOTES

SUPPLIES NEEDED	PURCHASED	DETAILS

SUMMARY OF DUTIES DONE & ANY CONCERNS

_____
_____
_____
_____
_____

CARE LOG

DATE		CARER	
START TIME		TIME ENDED	

MEDICATION	DOSE	TIME	NOTES

MEALS		TIME	QUANTITY
Breakfast			
Lunch			
Dinner			
Snack			
Snack			

TIME	ACTIVITIES	NAPS	TIME	TIME UP

PERSONAL HYGIENE	TIME	NOTES

SUPPLIES NEEDED	PURCHASED	DETAILS

SUMMARY OF DUTIES DONE & ANY CONCERNS

CARE LOG

DATE		CARER	
START TIME		TIME ENDED	

MEDICATION	DOSE	TIME	NOTES

MEALS		TIME	QUANTITY
Breakfast			
Lunch			
Dinner			
Snack			
Snack			

TIME	ACTIVITIES	NAPS	TIME	TIME UP

PERSONAL HYGIENE	TIME	NOTES

SUPPLIES NEEDED	PURCHASED	DETAILS

SUMMARY OF DUTIES DONE & ANY CONCERNS

CARE LOG

DATE		CARER	
START TIME		TIME ENDED	

MEDICATION	DOSE	TIME	NOTES

MEALS		TIME	QUANTITY
Breakfast			
Lunch			
Dinner			
Snack			
Snack			

TIME	ACTIVITIES	NAPS	TIME	TIME UP

PERSONAL HYGIENE	TIME	NOTES

SUPPLIES NEEDED	PURCHASED	DETAILS

SUMMARY OF DUTIES DONE & ANY CONCERNS

CARE LOG

DATE		CARER	
START TIME		TIME ENDED	

MEDICATION	DOSE	TIME	NOTES

MEALS		TIME	QUANTITY
Breakfast			
Lunch			
Dinner			
Snack			
Snack			

TIME	ACTIVITIES	NAPS	TIME	TIME UP

PERSONAL HYGIENE	TIME	NOTES

SUPPLIES NEEDED	PURCHASED	DETAILS

SUMMARY OF DUTIES DONE & ANY CONCERNS

_____
_____
_____
_____
_____

CARE LOG

DATE		CARER	
START TIME		TIME ENDED	

MEDICATION	DOSE	TIME	NOTES

MEALS		TIME	QUANTITY
Breakfast			
Lunch			
Dinner			
Snack			
Snack			

TIME	ACTIVITIES	NAPS	TIME	TIME UP

PERSONAL HYGIENE	TIME	NOTES

SUPPLIES NEEDED	PURCHASED	DETAILS

SUMMARY OF DUTIES DONE & ANY CONCERNS

CARE LOG

DATE		CARER	
START TIME		TIME ENDED	

MEDICATION	DOSE	TIME	NOTES

MEALS		TIME	QUANTITY
Breakfast			
Lunch			
Dinner			
Snack			
Snack			

TIME	ACTIVITIES	NAPS	TIME	TIME UP

PERSONAL HYGIENE	TIME	NOTES

SUPPLIES NEEDED	PURCHASED	DETAILS

SUMMARY OF DUTIES DONE & ANY CONCERNS

CARE LOG

DATE		CARER	
START TIME		TIME ENDED	

MEDICATION	DOSE	TIME	NOTES

MEALS		TIME	QUANTITY
Breakfast			
Lunch			
Dinner			
Snack			
Snack			

TIME	ACTIVITIES	NAPS	TIME	TIME UP

PERSONAL HYGIENE	TIME	NOTES

SUPPLIES NEEDED	PURCHASED	DETAILS

SUMMARY OF DUTIES DONE & ANY CONCERNS

CARE LOG

DATE		CARER	
START TIME		TIME ENDED	

MEDICATION	DOSE	TIME	NOTES

MEALS		TIME	QUANTITY
Breakfast			
Lunch			
Dinner			
Snack			
Snack			

TIME	ACTIVITIES	NAPS	TIME	TIME UP

PERSONAL HYGIENE	TIME	NOTES

SUPPLIES NEEDED	PURCHASED	DETAILS

SUMMARY OF DUTIES DONE & ANY CONCERNS

_____
_____
_____
_____
_____
_____

CARE LOG

DATE		CARER	
START TIME		TIME ENDED	

MEDICATION	DOSE	TIME	NOTES

MEALS		TIME	QUANTITY
Breakfast			
Lunch			
Dinner			
Snack			
Snack			

TIME	ACTIVITIES	NAPS	TIME	TIME UP

PERSONAL HYGIENE	TIME	NOTES

SUPPLIES NEEDED	PURCHASED	DETAILS

SUMMARY OF DUTIES DONE & ANY CONCERNS

CARE LOG

DATE		CARER	
START TIME		TIME ENDED	

MEDICATION	DOSE	TIME	NOTES

MEALS		TIME	QUANTITY
Breakfast			
Lunch			
Dinner			
Snack			
Snack			

TIME	ACTIVITIES	NAPS	TIME	TIME UP

PERSONAL HYGIENE	TIME	NOTES

SUPPLIES NEEDED	PURCHASED	DETAILS

SUMMARY OF DUTIES DONE & ANY CONCERNS

CARE LOG

DATE		CARER	
START TIME		TIME ENDED	

MEDICATION	DOSE	TIME	NOTES

MEALS		TIME	QUANTITY
Breakfast			
Lunch			
Dinner			
Snack			
Snack			

TIME	ACTIVITIES	NAPS	TIME	TIME UP

PERSONAL HYGIENE	TIME	NOTES

SUPPLIES NEEDED	PURCHASED	DETAILS

SUMMARY OF DUTIES DONE & ANY CONCERNS

CARE LOG

DATE		CARER	
START TIME		TIME ENDED	

MEDICATION	DOSE	TIME	NOTES

MEALS		TIME	QUANTITY
Breakfast			
Lunch			
Dinner			
Snack			
Snack			

TIME	ACTIVITIES	NAPS	TIME	TIME UP

PERSONAL HYGIENE	TIME	NOTES

SUPPLIES NEEDED	PURCHASED	DETAILS

SUMMARY OF DUTIES DONE & ANY CONCERNS

CARE LOG

DATE		CARER	
START TIME		TIME ENDED	

MEDICATION	DOSE	TIME	NOTES

MEALS		TIME	QUANTITY
Breakfast			
Lunch			
Dinner			
Snack			
Snack			

TIME	ACTIVITIES	NAPS	TIME	TIME UP

PERSONAL HYGIENE	TIME	NOTES

SUPPLIES NEEDED	PURCHASED	DETAILS

SUMMARY OF DUTIES DONE & ANY CONCERNS

CONTACT DETAILS

STAFF / AGENCY	CONTACT DETAILS

STAFF / AGENCY	CONTACT DETAILS

NOTES

NOTES

NOTES

NOTES

NOTES

NOTES

Made in the USA
Columbia, SC
20 November 2020

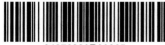
24976830R00065